Moto Medic

First Aid and Injury Prevention for Motorcyclists

Don Clutter

Order this book online at www.trafford.com/08-1430
or email orders@trafford.com

Most Trafford titles are also available at major online book retailers.

Note for Librarians: A cataloguing record for this book is available from Library
and Archives Canada at www.collectionscanada.ca/amicus/index-e.html

Printed in Victoria, BC, Canada.

ISBN: 978-1-4251-9019-4 (Soft)
ISBN: 978-1-4251-9021-7 (e-book)

*We at Trafford believe that it is the responsibility of us all, as both individuals
and corporations, to make choices that are environmentally and socially sound.
You, in turn, are supporting this responsible conduct each time you purchase a
Trafford book, or make use of our publishing services. To find out how you are
helping, please visit www.trafford.com/responsiblepublishing.html*

*Our mission is to efficiently provide the world's finest, most comprehensive
book publishing service, enabling every author to experience success.
To find out how to publish your book, your way, and have it available
worldwide, visit us online at www.trafford.com/10510*

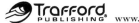 www.trafford.com

North America & international
toll-free: 1 888 232 4444 (USA & Canada)
phone: 250 383 6864 ♦ fax: 250 383 6804 ♦ email: info@trafford.com

The United Kingdom & Europe
phone: +44 (0)1865 487 395 ♦ local rate: 0845 230 9601
facsimile: +44 (0)1865 481 507 ♦ email: info.uk@trafford.com

10 9 8 7 6 5 4 3 2 1

CONTENTS

INTRODUCTION

MOTORCYCLING has many rewards, as those of us who ride can attest to. We also know only too well the risks associated with riding, and we readily accept those risks, hoping all the while that we and our friends never have to confront that particular demon. Occasionally, though, the devil raises his ugly head and bites one of us on the ass. Hopefully this manual will tell you how to put a band-aid on that bite.

IF we look at the three mechanisms of injury, i.e.: trauma, environmental, and medical; we can easily see that 'trauma' is of great concern to motorcyclists. It may not be as readily apparent, but if we think about the environmental factors that motorcyclists are exposed to, we will realize that environmental mechanisms of injury are equally important to motorcyclists.

THERE are many excellent first-aid manuals available, but most of those will include a lot of good information we don't usually need and may not have something we will need if and when that time comes. A first-aid manual geared toward motorcyclists can provide the specific tools needed to effectively deal with the most common injuries and conditions motorcyclists face. Ideally, the information in this manual should be supplemented with a CPR class and a first-aid class with hands-on practice that would help

1

familiarize people with the information and make them more comfortable using it when they need it. We can never be too prepared when it comes to our well-being and safety.

WHEN riding solo it is important to have this information and a good first aid kit available because you may be the only one around for a considerable amount of time to provide any aid in case of an accident or injury to yourself. Every group of friends or club that has group rides should have at least one person familiar with first aid and CPR and have at least one good first aid kit along on every group ride.

THE information in this manual can also help motorcyclists avoid situations that lead to accidents or prevent their resultant injuries. Unfortunately, many motorcyclists unwittingly or negligently do things that contribute to their risk. It is good to know how to treat an injury effectively, but it is better to know how to avoid an accident or prevent an injury from happening.

RIDE HARD.   RIDE SAFE.   BE PREPARED.

PART 1

INJURY PREVENTION

THE best way to treat an injury is to prevent it. There are many things a motorcyclist can do to prevent or at least reduce the severity of both injuries and the accidents that cause them. For many the "cost" of the prevention doesn't seem worth it to them – for instance, how many motorcyclists will give up their black leather jackets for a bright yellow one that is much more conspicuous to oblivious car drivers? How many would cover their cut-off T-shirts with <u>any</u> jacket on hot days? Since individual choice in our level of risk is one of the inherent attractions in motorcycling, each person has to decide for themselves what preventive measures they will take and what risks they will assume - just remember you made certain choices when you're picking gravel out of that nasty road rash.

THE number of single-vehicle motorcycle accidents has been steadily climbing and it will take a well-funded comprehensive research study to figure out all the reasons why, but until that happens I'm going to offer my two cents worth. I believe a significant number of those accidents and the accompanying injuries could have easily been avoided with a little preventive action. For instance, many of the conditions addressed in this book (dehydration, hypothermia, altitude sickness, etc.) first manifest themselves as a decrease in mental acuity. This means if you are riding in 95 degree weather wearing a cut-off T-shirt and you had a beer or cup of coffee at that last stop instead of water, the reason you didn't make that turn and plowed into the telephone pole may be because you were experiencing the first stages of dehydration and not just because you are a poor rider. If you live at the beach and you are on your first ride over a 10,000 foot mountain pass in the Rockies, the reason you didn't brake soon enough and ran into that slow moving 18 wheeler might be because your judgment was impaired by the onset of altitude sickness. I will also say that if you're riding on Angeles Crest and you chopped the throttle and hit the brakes when you felt a little too hot in that corner and hi-sided over the cliff, it might be because you skipped that cornering class your buddy asked you to go to. Proper instruction can help you become a better rider and avoid accidents regardless how long you've been riding.

- o **BELOW** is a list of things that will contribute to preventing accidents and injuries, or will help in reducing the severity of injuries in case you do have an accident. You may agree or disagree with these suggestions, but, again, it is up to each individual rider to decide for themselves and make their own decisions.

o **Wear a helmet**. OK, if you're one of the black-clad clone army, let me say this first – I think everyone over the age of 18 should be able to decide for themselves if they want to wear a helmet or not. That said, anyone who decides not to wear a helmet deserves to have pudding for a brain if you bonk your noggin. A helmet does not help prevent accidents - you are as likely as not to have an accident if you wear one - but it definitely does help lessen the severity of head injuries in cases of non-fatal accidents. In many fatal accidents, but not all, there are usually enough other potentially fatal injuries that the person would die irrespective of their head injury (Indian Larry, who would most probably not be dead from a very minor accident if he had been wearing a helmet, is one of the notable exceptions). A full-face helmet offers the most protection, but an open-faced helmet is better than a beanie and much better than nothing. Research has shown that a helmet does <u>not</u> impair your vision or hearing at riding speeds. Also, anyone who says a helmet contributes to injuries rather than lessens them is uninformed, misinformed, or just plain ignorant and should read the research.

o **Learn how to ride better**. Everyone can be a better rider than they are, no matter how long they have been riding. With all of the different instruction available out there, there is no reason not to take advantage of someone else's expertise. Take a dirt bike class to learn how to handle loss of traction; or a street class to learn about counter-steering, how to use your brakes most effectively, not chopping the throttle in a turn, or any of the other million skills necessary to ride well. Then go out and really practice the things you learn. In the appendix there is a list of suggestions for some excellent skills improvement classes.

o **Be conspicuous**. Things like headlight modulators and louder horns can aid greatly in being conspicuous, but, no, loud pipes do not save lives, they only annoy people. Every motorcycle rider I know, as well as every car driver, has had the experience while driving their car of having a motorcycle come up beside them and surprise them because they couldn't hear the motorcycle, no matter how loud, until the motorcycle went past them because the sound is directed behind the motorcycle. That car that's going to turn left in front of you will not hear your loud pipes, (unless your exhaust faces forward) and probably will not see you unless you do something to visually draw their attention, which has been shown in research to be the most effective way of being conspicuous. Wearing bright colored clothing and helmets will definitely help in that respect – the question is how far will you go in abandoning fashion for a little more safety?

o **Don't drink (or use drugs) and ride.** The two most common factors in single-vehicle motorcycle accidents are alcohol and excessive speed. Obviously, motorcyclists need all of their faculties at peak performance. Even if you are one of those people who think that their reactions are better after a drink or two, there are other reasons not to. Alcohol can contribute to conditions like dehydration and the combined reduction in mental acuity from the alcohol and the onset of dehydration can reduce your judgment enough to get you into a bad situation you otherwise wouldn't be in. Even prescription or over the counter drugs can dull reactions and mental acuity enough to contribute to an accident.

o **Don't ride faster than the conditions or your skill level will safely allow.** As stated above, excessive speed is one of the biggest factors associated with single-vehicle motorcycle accidents. 'Excessive speed' doesn't just mean what is posted on the sign, it also means faster than you are capable of safely going given your skill level and the conditions you are riding in. Butt-puckering is one of the best early-warning indicators that you are going too fast.   Pay attention when your butt tells you something.

o **Wear protective gear.** The most obvious advantage to wearing good riding gear will be in helping to keep the rider's skin and body parts where they belong in case of a get-off.   Wear good boots with padding or hard protection in the ankles, toes, and heels rather than tennis shoes. Riding pants with armor, padding, or Kevlar in the knees, hips, and tailbone area are almost as good as a fully armored leather racing suit. At the least wear heavy denim long pants, never shorts.   Wear good gloves. The ones with hard armor over the knuckles, extra padding in the palms and secure fasteners over the wrists are best, but elk skin ropers are way better than nothing.   Additionally, wearing the right gear can help immensely in reducing the negative effects of the environment and in staving off life-threatening situations. For example, you may think that wearing your Harley T-shirt with the sleeves cut off while riding in 100 degree weather through the Mojave Desert on your way to Laughlin makes you cooler, but the truth is it's a good way to open the door for dehydration, heat exhaustion, or heat stroke. It is much better, and much more comfortable, to wear a properly designed well-ventilated motorcycle jacket, especially if you wear one of those microfiber cooling vests that you soak in water underneath your well-ventilated jacket. This will keep your core temperature at a very comfortable and very safe level. Wearing a long-sleeved blue cotton work shirt over your cut-off T-shirt in cold conditions might look biker-cool, but it won't do much for preventing hypothermia.

o **Be aware of your mental state.** Many motorcyclists, if not most, use riding as a way to clear out the cobwebs, sort out the crap buzzing around their brain, or just to get a clearer and calmer perspective on things. If your mental state is distracting you from the task at hand (riding well), pull over and sit it out a while or postpone that ride until you can devote the proper concentration to it.

o **Keep up on the maintenance of your bike.** While you are speeding down a nice twisty road is not a good time to find out that all the bolts holding your front wheel on have come loose, your brake fluid reservoir is empty, and that your rear tire pressure is down to 18 pounds. Check your bike, all of the fluid levels, and the tire pressures before every ride.

o **Read this book.** Take it and your first aid kit on every ride. Take a CPR class.

ACCIDENT SCENE MANAGEMENT

FIRST, secure the scene. Put out flares if anyone has them. If they are available, post people at each end of the accident scene to stop or slow oncoming vehicles and direct traffic around victims, fuel or oil spills, downed motorcycles, debris, etc. to prevent further accidents and additional injuries. If no one is available to direct traffic, move victims who can't move themselves off of the roadway. Unconscious victims or those with suspected head/cervical/spinal injuries must be carefully moved to prevent further injury. The best way to accomplish this is to kneel above the victim's head using your forearms under their head and neck while grasping their shoulders, jacket, shirt, etc. and dragging them by pulling towards the head (see photos below). Move vehicles or large debris away as soon as possible.

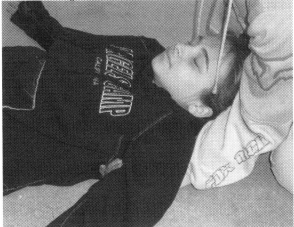

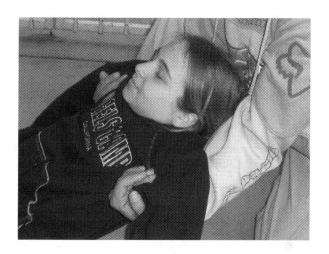

NEXT, evaluate the injuries. Determine if the injuries are minor, requiring only first aid; or major, requiring immediate intervention &/or emergency medical attention. Pay particular attention to shock and possible internal, head, and cervical/spinal injuries, which can be life threatening and are frequently minimized by the victims, who may express that they are OK when they are not. All motorcycle accident victims should be considered as possible candidates for head, neck/spinal, and internal injuries. If there are major injuries or if there is any question at all, emergency medical services (EMS) should be called immediately.

DETERMINE if anyone needs CPR or other immediate attention, such as for severe bleeding, and provide that aid. If the person is unconscious, unless they need CPR or are bleeding uncontrollably from a head or face wound, <u>leave their helmet on.</u> The emergency medical personnel will want to take it off themselves and will want to see the location and type of specific damages to help evaluate underlying injuries. Only remove a helmet if absolutely necessary to provide CPR or other critical aid.

IF it is necessary to remove the helmet, the best method to do so requires two people (see photos on pages 13-14). One person should be at the side of the head and the other directly above the head of the victim (see photos A and C). Glasses or sunglasses should be removed and please remember to unbuckle the chinstrap. The person at the side should have one hand at the base of the skull (not on the helmet) and one hand on the chin or jaw (again, not on the helmet) to stabilize the victim's head. The person behind the victim's head should pull the helmet slowly and directly back (photo D), or roll it off back and up if it is a full face helmet (photo B). When the helmet is off, something should be placed under the head, such as a rolled-up shirt or jacket, to help stabilize the person's head.

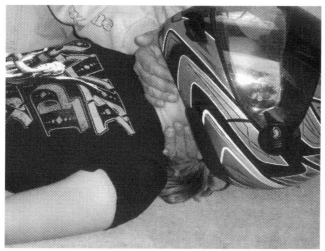

Photo A

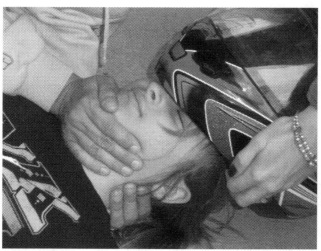

Photo B

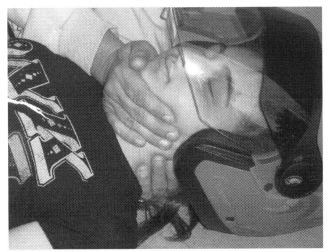

Photo C

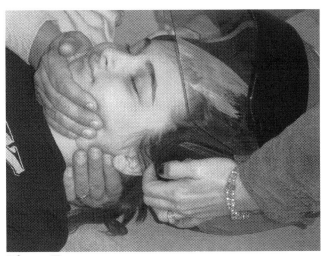

Photo D

CALL for emergency medical services immediately if needed. Remember that cell phone calls to 911 do not necessarily go to the closest dispatcher; they usually are routed to regional dispatch centers which can greatly increase the time necessary in answering the call and in responding to it. Cell phones also don't show the dispatcher where the calls are originating from. Cell phone service is not always available in all locations. Land-line calls are best if they are readily available because they go to the nearest dispatcher and show the location of the call. If no cell phone service is available, someone will need to leave the accident scene to make the call. In either case, make sure the caller knows the exact location of the accident scene. The caller should also know how many victims there are, and, to the best of their ability, the condition of each victim. The caller should wait for the 911 Operator to hang up first; the caller hangs up last. Keep in mind that more than one ambulance might be required if there is more than one injured person, and be sure to let the dispatcher know this.

WHEN emergency medical services personnel arrive give them a factual account of the accident – exactly what happened, how fast they were going, who hit who or what, and if it is known if any drugs or alcohol were involved. If the information can be obtained from the victims, EMS personnel need to know of any allergies, any medical conditions or medications, and what and when did they last eat or drink anything. Also important information is what steps, if any, have been taken by the people on scene. Give EMS personnel the time and space they need to do their job. Be aware that EMS personnel will cut helmet straps and cut off leather jackets or other clothes. <u>Don't freak out – these things can be replaced - let them do their job.</u>

EMERGENCY Information Cards are a good idea for everyone to carry. These should have emergency contact information, any medical conditions or alerts, any medications, and any allergies, especially medication allergies. If you carry one of these in your wallet or pocket, let someone know it is there so this information can be used if needed. To hold emergency information in a more obvious place, there are small pouches that attach to the helmet or helmet strap available for this purpose.

I travel not to go anywhere, but to go. I travel for travel's sake. The great affair is to move.

Robert Louis Stevenson

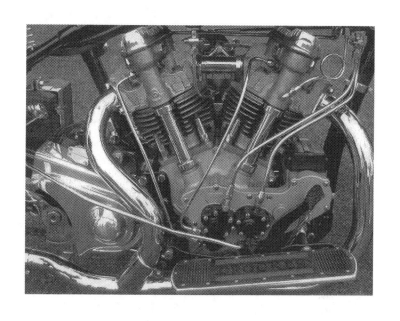

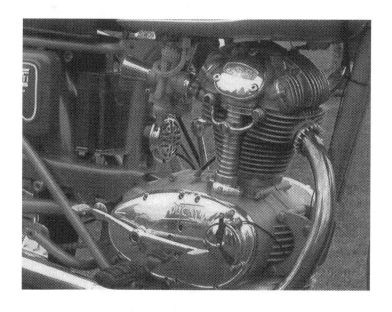

PART 2

ENVIRONMENTAL FACTORS

THERE are many things in the environment that we ride through that are potential sources of injury for motorcyclists other than the things we run into or that run into us. The weather itself can present life-threatening situations for us to deal with. Dust, dirt, rocks, insects, or other small objects whizzing by are all potential sources of injury, as are the many hot, sharp, and heavy objects on our bikes themselves. Even the zippers on our jackets can inflict excruciating pain. Just sitting in the saddle can cause a case of Monkey-Butt that can ruin even the best ride. It can be a cruel and hostile world out there.

ENVIRONMENTAL factors can also have indirect dire consequences. Dehydration, heat exhaustion, heat stroke, hypothermia, and altitude sickness can all begin with a decrease in mental acuity and functioning. Combine this with a little alcohol, too much coffee, or sleep deprivation and the resultant decrease in judgment can contribute to making bad decisions that lead to an accident causing major injuries or death. No one really knows how many single-vehicle motorcycle accidents or motorcycle vs. other vehicle accidents have had these simple environmental factors contributing to a rider's decreased awareness or acuity which then leads to an accident.

AN awareness of all the environmental factors affecting motorcyclists can be the first step in effectively preventing many of these emergencies. Knowing how to deal with these common environmental occurrences that can range from simply irritating to life-threatening can greatly enhance and extend our riding pleasure.

Riding a motorcycle on today's highways you have to ride in a very defensive way. You have to be a good rider and you have to have both hands and both feet on the controls at all times.

Evel Knievel

HYPOTHERMIA

HYPOTHERMIA occurs when the body cannot generate enough heat to replace what is lost through exposure to cold temperatures or a cool, damp environment and the body's core temperature drops below 95 degrees.

SIGNS and symptoms:
- o Shivering
- o Slurred speech
- o Slow breathing
- o Cold, pale skin
- o Loss of coordination
- o Fatigue, lethargy, apathy
- o Unaware of gradual loss of mental acuity & physical ability

DO:
- o Move out of cold and wind
- o Move indoors if possible
- o Cover the head – a large percentage of heat loss is through the head
- o Remove wet clothing and replace with warm dry clothing or other covering if available
- o Apply warm compresses to neck, chest, and groin areas
- o Summon emergency medical services immediately if breathing becomes excessively slow or shallow

o   Warm slowly and gently – the person is at risk for cardiac arrest

DON'T:
- o   **Apply dire: t heat, hot water, heating pad, et: .**
- o   **Attempt to warm arms & legs – heat applied to arms & legs for: es : old blood ba: k to the heart, lungs, & brain**
- o   **Give al: ohol**
- o   **Give hot drinks – only warm drinks**
- o   **Massage or rub : old body parts**
- o   **Smoke – it de: reases blood flow**

Avoiding danger is not safer in the long run than outright exposure. Life is either a daring adventure, or nothing.

Helen Keller

FROSTBITE

EXPOSURE to very cold temperatures, especially with wind, can freeze the skin and underlying tissue. The hands, feet, nose, and ears are most vulnerable.

SIGNS and symptoms:
- o Skin appears white and soft in superficial frostbite
- o Hard, pale, cold skin means a more serious frostbite
- o Skin becomes red and painful as it thaws
- o Deeper frostbite can produce blisters within 24 hours

DO:
- o Get out of the cold and into a warm area
- o Protect from wind
- o Warm hands by tucking under the arms
- o Warm hands or feet if indoors with warm, not hot, water
- o Warm nose, ears, or face by covering with dry gloved hands or other dry cloth
- o If already thawed, wrap up and warm to prevent refreezing
- o Get emergency medical treatment as soon as possible

DON'T:

- o Rub or massage area
- o Rub snow or i: e on area
- o Thaw out the frozen area if there is a : han: e of refreezing
- o Apply heating pads or hot water
- o Smoke – : auses vaso: onstri: tion and further de: reases blood flow

"Life is not a journey to the grave with the intention of arriving safely in a pretty and well-preserved body, but rather to skid in broadside, totally worn out and proclaiming, 'WOW, WHAT A RIDE!!!'"

Anonymous

ALTITUDE SICKNESS

THE effects of altitude sickness can begin between 8,000 and 10,000 feet. Failure to effectively address the early symptoms of altitude sickness can lead to the potentially fatal conditions of high altitude pulmonary or cerebral edema. Being young &/or in good physical condition does not reduce the risk of altitude sickness.

SIGNS and symptoms:
- o   Decrease in mental acuity
- o   Lack of coordination
- o   Headache
- o   Lethargy
- o   Dizziness
- o   Nausea
- o   Vomiting
- o   Difficulty breathing
- o   Bluish skin & nails
- o   Frequent coughing
- o   Frothy or pink sputum
- o   Irrational behavior
- o   Inability to sit up or walk

DO:
- o   Descend to lower altitude
- o   Avoid smoking or drinking alcohol
- o   Seek immediate emergency medical attention if any symptoms appear severe
- o   Rest an extra day for each 3,000 feet of altitude

- o Increase fluid intake prior to ascension
- o See your doctor prior to a ride to high altitudes about prescribing acetazolamide or dexamethasone

DON'T:
- o **As: end any higher until symptoms subside**
- o **Drink al: ohol**
- o **Smoke**

Most motorcycle problems are caused by the nut that connects the handlebars to the seat.

Anonymous

INSECT STINGS

BEE, wasp, hornet, and yellow jacket stings are common occurrences for motorcyclists and can range from a mild irritation to a life threatening condition. The insect venom triggers an immune reaction, the severity of which depends upon your sensitivity to the venom. Only a small percentage of people develop anaphylaxis, the most severe reaction.

SIGNS and symptoms:
- o Itching
- o Stinging
- o Fever
- o Swelling at the sting site, serious if over 2 inches in diameter
- o Hives, painful joints, swollen glands
- o Swelling of the lips & throat or other facial swelling
- o Difficulty breathing
- o Faintness or dizziness
- o Nausea, cramps, or diarrhea
- o Confusion, difficulty thinking clearly
- o Rapid heartbeat

DO:
- o Move to an area away from insects to avoid more stings
- o Scrape off stinger with credit card, back of knife, etc.
- o Apply ice or cold pack

- o Apply calamine lotion, Benadryl cream, or hydrocortisone cream
- o Take an antihistamine containing Benadryl
- o If allergic to stings, check if person has Epi-pen or other medication
- o Seek emergency medical attention if any indications of a severe reaction or any breathing difficulty
- o Treat for shock

DON'T:
- o **Try grabbing the stinger with fingers or tweezers to pull it out – that : an inje: t more venom into the person**
- o **Drink anything**

Four wheels moves the body, two wheels moves the soul.

Anonymous

ANAPHYLAXIS

ANAPHYLAXIS is a severe allergic reaction to something you breathe, swallow, or touch that can be fatal. Medicines, insect stings, foods, and latex are common things that can trigger a life-threatening allergic reaction. Symptoms usually appear quickly, within minutes of exposure, but can be delayed as long as 12 to 24 hours. Many people are not aware of their sensitivity until they have a severe reaction to something.

SIGNS and symptoms:
- o Difficulty breathing
- o Coughing or wheezing
- o Dizziness or fainting
- o Rapid or weak heartbeat
- o Swelling in the mouth or throat
- o Flushing, itching, or hives
- o Vomiting, diarrhea, or stomach cramps

DO:
- o Look for a medical alert tag that says what the person is allergic to
- o If the person is aware of their allergy, they may have injectable epinephrine with them, such as Epi-pen Auto Injection
- o Give epinephrine injection if the person has it
- o Give antihistamine
- o Call for Emergency Medical Services immediately

DON'T:
- o **Wait to : all EMS – do it as soon as there is any breathing diffi: ulty**

Wandering re-establishes the original harmony which once existed between man and the universe.

Anatole France

ZIPPER SNAGS

ANYONE with a zipper has gotten something caught in it at least once in their life, and wishes they hadn't. Aside from the usual much-feared male snag, big bellies and big zippers result in snagged belly buttons with alarming frequency. With the numerous heavy-duty zippers on men's and women's motorcycle gear our risks are even more pronounced.

SIGNS and symptoms:
- o Skin & possibly clothing caught in the teeth or between the teeth and slide of a zipper
- o Pain
- o Bleeding

DO:
- o Try lubricating with mineral oil & <u>gently</u> manipulating the zipper
- o If mineral oil doesn't work, cut the zipper slide with wire cutters or metal snips as shown in the illustration – be careful what you cut
- o After cutting the slide, gently separate the zipper teeth
- o Cleanse the affected area thoroughly to prevent infection
- o Apply antibiotic ointment and cover loosely with a non-stick dressing

DON'T:
- o Cut : lothing or skin – only the zipper
- o Yank : lothing & skin out of the snag

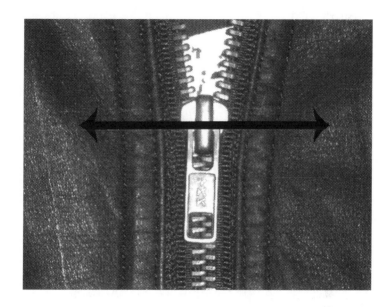

FRICTION BLISTERS

FRICTION blisters are from unprotected skin rubbing against something. For motorcyclists friction blisters appear most frequently on the feet or hands from using new boots or equipment without proper break-in prior to a ride. To help prevent blisters on the feet, apply an antiperspirant containing aluminum chloride to the feet beginning at least three days prior to a ride and use good athletic or riding socks with extra padding in critical areas.

SIGNS and symptoms:
- o Open or intact blister
- o Pain
- o Difficulty walking if they are on the feet

DO:
- o If blister is intact, cover with protective dressing like gauze and tape or band-aid or cover the blister with Second Skin or Dermabond then cover with padding
- o If blister is torn or broken open, apply antibiotic ointment and cover with non-stick bandage
- o Attach Moleskin to inside of shoes at friction points

DON'T:
- o **Break open or drain blister**
- o **Remove skin : overing blister if it is drained**

Everyone crashes. Some get back on. Some don't. Some can't.

Anonymous

FOREIGN OBJECT IN THE SKIN

MINOR impalements of foreign objects in the skin are frequent occurrences that unfortunately are many times made worse rather than better by the wrong interventions.

SIGNS and symptoms:
- o Small slivers of wood, metal, plastic, fiberglass, or other material embedded in or projecting from the skin
- o Pain and sometimes minor bleeding

DO:
- o If projecting from the skin with little or no bleeding, use sterilized tweezers to remove
- o If completely embedded, use sterilized needle to gently lift out the tip of the object, then remove with sterilized tweezers
- o After the object is removed, clean the area well and apply antibiotic ointment
- o If a large object is embedded in someone or driven completely through a limb or if there is excessive bleeding, stabilize the object and get immediate emergency medical attention

DON'T:
- o **Try to squeeze out or push out the obje:t**
- o **Try to remove any large obje:ts embedded in someone, :ompletely through a limb, or if there is ex:essive bleeding**

I soon realized that no journey carries one far unless, as it extends into the world around us, it goes an equal distance into the world within.

Lillian Smith

FOREIGN OBJECT IN THE NOSE

MOTORCYCLISTS ride through an environment with many foreign objects like insects or small rocks that can become lodged in places they don't belong, like various bodily orifices. Since our nose leads the way, it is one of the most common places to get things in that we want out.

SIGNS and symptoms:
- o Something in your nose that doesn't belong there
- o Pain or discomfort
- o Difficulty breathing through that nostril

DO:
- o Breathe through the mouth until the object is removed
- o Close the other nostril and breathe <u>out gently</u> through the blocked nostril
- o If the object is visible and can be easily grasped with tweezers without pushing in farther, gently remove
- o Seek medical attention if unable to remove

DON'T:

- o Probe for an unseen obje:t with finger, q-tip, tool, or other devi: e
- o Breathe in through the nose for: efully
- o Blow your nose hard or repeatedly

A good traveler has no fixed plans, and is not intent upon arriving.

Lao Tzu

FOREIGN OBJECT IN EAR

ANOTHER common place motorcyclists find foreign objects are the ears. Insects seem to especially like crawling into this warm dark spot.

SIGNS and symptoms:
- o Something that doesn't belong there stuck in your ear
- o Pain or discomfort
- o Difficulty hearing

DO:
- o If you can see the object and it can be easily grasped with tweezers without pushing it in farther, gently remove it
- o Tilt the head with the affected side down, gently shake to try to dislodge the object
- o Position the head with the effected ear up and try floating it out with mineral oil (best thing to do if it is a live or dead insect)
- o If unable to remove or symptoms persist, seek medical attention

DON'T:
- o Probe for unseen obje:t with q-tip, tool, et:.
- o Use mineral oil if there is dis:harge or bleeding
- o Use mineral oil if you suspe:t a perforated eardrum
- o Slap or pound on the other ear – it will only hurt your other ear

Half the fun of travel is the esthetic of lostness.

Ray Bradbury

FOREIGN OBJECT IN THE EYE

THE importance of always wearing eye protection for motorcyclists cannot be stressed enough. The eye is fragile and our chosen activity puts them at risk every time we ride. If you can't wear a helmet with a good shield at least always wear good eye protection with shatterproof lenses.

SIGNS and symptoms:
- o Something in the eye causing watering, redness, repeated blinking, or pain

DO:
- o If the object is floating on the surface of the eye, try gently flushing it out with saline solution or clean lukewarm water
- o Use an eyewash kit if you have one in your first aid kit
- o If the pain persists after the object is flushed out, get emergency medical assistance
- o If the object does not flush out or is embedded in the eye, get emergency medical assistance
- o If the pain persists after the object is flushed out, get emergency medical assistance
- o If the embedded object is large enough to make closing the eye difficult, cover the

eye with an eye cup, a Styrofoam cup, or a paper cup

DON'T:
- o **Try to remove an obje:t embedded in the eyeball**
- o **Try to get the obje:t out of the eye by rubbing**

No one realizes how beautiful it is to travel until he comes home and rests his head on his old, familiar pillow.

Lin Yutang

DISLOCATED CONTACT LENS

EVEN when wearing a full-face helmet with a faceshield contact lenses can get blown out of the eye or displaced. In addition to being uncomfortable or painful, a displaced contact lens obviously makes safe riding difficult.

SIGNS and symptoms:
- o   Pain or watering from a contact lens being blown or rubbed out of place
- o   Impaired vision from a missing lens

DO:
- o   Pull back the eyelid and rotate the eye to try to locate the lens
- o   If the lens is dislocated and visible, gently slide it over the cornea
- o   Have the person then remove it as usual – some people have a rubber suction cup for removing hard lenses or a soft rubber tweezer-like device for removing soft lenses
- o   Treat any corneal abrasions as described in that section
- o   If the lens cannot be located, it may be in the deepest recess under the upper lid and may be floated out by using the eye wash kit in your first aid kit, or
- o   Try to float it out by gently flooding with saline solution or clean lukewarm water

DON'T:
- o **Give up if you : an't see the lens, it : an be out of sight behind the eyeball**
- o **Irritate or injure the eye by poking and prodding with fingers or q-tips, et: – sometimes there is no lens to be found**

I have found that there ain't no surer way to find out whether you like people or hate them than to travel with them.

Mark Twain

CORNEAL ABRASION

THE lens of the eye can be scratched by sand, dirt, dust, or other windblown detritus. Dry eyes are also very susceptible to scratching from rubbing. A corneal abrasion can become a serious eye problem if not treated quickly and effectively.

SIGNS and symptoms:
- o   Tears
- o   Blurred vision
- o   Redness
- o   A feeling like sand in the eyes
- o   Pain

DO:
- o   Check for an object in the eye causing the scratch, treat as described in "Foreign Object In The Eye"
- o   Rinse out the eye with saline solution or clean lukewarm water, or
- o   Use the eyewash kit in your first aid kit
- o   Seek medical attention as soon as possible to prevent infection of the eye

DON'T:
- o   **Apply i: e pa: ks or pat: hes**
- o   **Aggravate the injury by rubbing**

BURNS – MINOR

WHAT distinguishes a minor burn from a serious burn is the extent of tissue damage. In a first – degree burn only the outer layer of skin is burned, but hasn't been burned through.

SIGNS and symptoms:
- o Dry, reddened skin
- o Minor swelling
- o Pain
- o No blisters

DO:
- o Cool the area by holding it under cool running water
- o If running water is not available, immerse the area in cool water or
- o Apply a cold compress
- o Watch for signs of infection
- o Use sunscreen on burned area
- o Take over-the-counter pain relievers

DON'T:
- o **Put i: e on the burned area**
- o **Tan the burned area for at least a year**
- o **Re-injure or allow the area to sunburn**

BURNS – SECOND DEGREE

SECOND – DEGREE burns are when the first layer of skin (epidermis) has been burned through and the second layer (dermis) is burned. Second – degree burns on the face, hands, feet, groin, buttocks, over a major joint, or more than 3 inches in diameter are more serious.

SIGNS and symptoms:
- o Red, splotchy appearance
- o Blisters
- o Severe pain
- o Swelling

DO:
- o Cool the area by holding it under cool running water until the pain subsides
- o If running water is not available, immerse the area in cool water
- o Apply cold compresses
- o Apply aloe vera lotion or antibiotic ointment once cooled
- o Cover with loose sterile gauze bandage
- o Watch for signs of infection
- o Take over-the-counter pain relievers

DON'T:
- o   **Break blisters**
- o   **Use i: e – : an : ause frostbite**
- o   **Use fluffy : otton - : an irritate the skin**
- o   **Put any pressure on the burned skin**
- o   **Re-injure or sunburn the area**

It is not down in any map: true places never are.

Herman Melville

BURNS – THIRD DEGREE

THE most serious burns involve all layers of the skin. Fat, muscle, or even bone may be affected. Third – degree burns are serious and emergency medical assistance should be summoned.

SIGNS and symptoms:
- o Skin may appear charred black or dry and white
- o Burned area may be deep into tissue
- o Usually painless
- o May be second – degree burns and blisters around burn area

DO:
- o Make sure there is no burning or smoldering material still in contact with the person
- o Check for breathing and circulation
- o Cover the burned area with moist sterile bandage or clean moist cloth or towel
- o Call for emergency medical assistance immediately

DON'T:
- o **Remove already burnt : lothing**
- o **Immerse severe burns in water – : ould : ause sho: k**
- o **Apply any ointment or lotions**

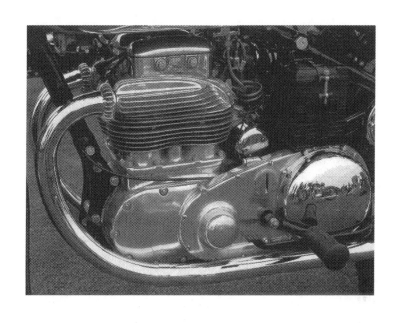

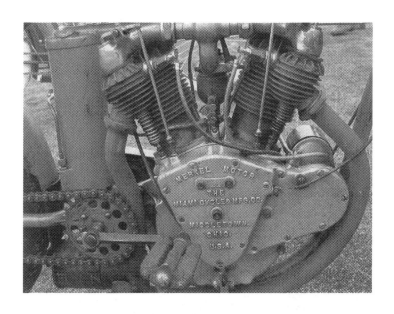

MONKEY BUTT

WHETHER you call it Monkey Butt, jock itch, or seat rash, it isn't very pleasant and can easily ruin even the best ride. It is caused by fungus and brought on by moisture, warmth, and friction. Unfortunately, what may start as a fungal infection may be made worse by an allergic reaction to the soap, shampoo, or detergent you use, or even the cream or ointment you apply to cure the Monkey Butt. This is one place where an ounce of prevention really is better than a pound of cure.

SIGNS and symptoms:
- o Can be uncomfortable to very painful
- o Red, raised rash in groin area
- o Itchy
- o Red wet rash could mean a possible Candida infection
- o Burning sensation or blistering can indicate allergic reaction

DO:
- o Clean and dry the area well
- o Apply an antifungal like Tinactin, Desenex, Lotrimin, Micatin, or
- o Apply Balmex or Desitin (yes, the diaper rash stuff you used on your children) or
- o Apply a powder like Anti Monkey Butt Powder as a drying agent
- o Take oral antihistamines if allergic reaction

- o To prevent it:
    - o Shower daily & wear clean underwear
    - o Keep the area dry and clean
    - o Avoid clothes that chafe (try those tight bicycling or motorcycling shorts – they really do work)

DON'T:
- o **Start using any new detergents, soaps, et: right before a ride**
- o **Use tal: um powder**
- o **Wear :lothes tha t :haf e**
- o **Keep using a : ream, ointment, or powder if the rash gets worse (: ould be an allergi: rea:tion)**
- o **Use steroid : reams (: ortisone) or antihistamine lotions (Benadryl)**
- o **Use : ombination antifungal and steroid : reams (Lotrisone or My: olog)**

PART 3

HEAT DISORDERS

HEAT disorders are some of the most common and most dangerous environmental risks that motorcyclists face. They are also the most insidious due to the fact that many motorcyclists do not recognize the onset of heat disorders while unknowingly doing things that contribute to heat related emergencies. Additionally, the first effects of some heat disorders are a decrease in mental acuity and a difficulty thinking clearly. An impending heat disorder combined with a pre-existing medical condition and some unwitting contributory actions by a motorcyclist can result in a decrease in reaction time, coordination, or judgment that leads to an accident. The underlying causes of many motorcycle accidents may prove to be linked to the overlooked effects of heat disorders.

HEAT related emergencies can happen to otherwise healthy, fit individuals. Heat disorders occur when body temperatures rise above normal or when the body loses its ability to effectively regulate heat. Dehydration can be the first warning sign in impending heat related emergencies and is an early step in the heat disorder continuum. It is also a contributing factor in more serious heat related emergencies. Dehydration is a decrease in the body's fluid level below what is required for adequate circulation caused by excessive perspiration, vomiting, or diarrhea with inadequate fluid intake to replace what has been lost.

HEAT exhaustion is the next step beyond dehydration in the heat disorder continuum. Heat exhaustion usually occurs after repeated periods over several days of heat exposure and fluid loss with inadequate fluid replacement. As blood flow to the vital organs decreases due to the fluid loss a form of shock sets in which can result in a drop in blood pressure, circulatory collapse, and unconsciousness.

IF heat exhaustion is not treated quickly and effectively it can progress to heat stroke (or sunstroke), which is less common but much more serious. Heat stroke is a life-threatening situation and calls for immediate emergency medical attention. Heat stroke occurs when the body's heat regulating mechanisms fail and the body's temperature rises. When the body generates more heat than it can dissipate, this heat accumulates, raising the body's core temperature. Core temperature can rise to the point of causing widespread physiological dysfunction leading to brain or other vital organ damage and death.

THERE are many factors that can contribute to heat disorders and heat related emergencies.

Some of the following conditions can increase vulnerability to heat disorders, inhibit the production of sweat, or interfere with the efficient evaporation of sweat. Sweating is the body's most important mechanism for heat dissipation.

- o Decreased physical fitness
- o Excessive body weight
- o Lack of sleep – less than 5 hours per night
- o Poor circulation
- o Inefficient sweat glands
- o Sunburns – interferes with body's heat regulation
- o Consumption of alcohol
- o Consumption of caffeinated drinks
- o Eating high fat foods
- o Eating high sodium foods

COMMON over-the-counter, prescription, and street drugs can contribute to heat related emergencies. Some impair the body's ability to regulate heat. Others slow sweat production or restrict blood flow to the skin which impedes the body's ability to release heat. Some increase fluid loss, upsetting the body's fluid balance. Some drugs to be especially careful with are:

- o Diuretics
- o Sedatives
- o Anti-depressants
- o Tranquilizers
- o Anticholinergics
- o Antihistamines
- o Cardio-vascular drugs, especially vasoconstrictors & beta blockers

o Street drugs, especially hallucinogens, cocaine, & amphetamines, which increase muscle activity and body heat

CHRONIC medical conditions can increase a person's vulnerability to heat disorders or compound the effects creating a more serious heat related emergency. Some common conditions to be especially careful of are:
o Heart, lung, or kidney diseases
o High blood pressure
o Low blood pressure
o Diabetes
o Metabolic disorders
o Conditions requiring salt-restricted diets

PROPER hydration is critical in the prevention of heat disorders and heat related emergencies. Motorcyclists should be well hydrated prior to beginning a ride in warm and humid or hot weather. Don't wait until you are thirsty to hydrate – by then it is already too late. Drinking at least one quart of water every hour you are riding in hot weather is minimal. Continuous hydration using a hydration pack or other device is a much better way to stay hydrated. Proper riding gear aids greatly in avoiding heat related emergencies. The more exposed skin you have, the more vulnerable you are to dehydration and other heat related conditions. Cool water is the best for replacing lost fluid; caffeinated drinks or alcohol are the worst. Sweetened drinks should not be used since they impair the transit of water from the stomach to the small intestine, where the absorption of water occurs. Drinks with sugar or salt suppress the sense of thirst and so should be avoided. Non-carbonated sports drinks like Gatorade are OK. You do not want to take salt tablets, which may be more detrimental than helpful. A normal diet has enough salt reserve to meet that need.

REMEMBER, the more preventive action you take here the fewer emergencies you will have to deal with later.

Take any road you please... it curves always, which is a continual promise, whereas straight roads reveal everything at a glance and kill interest.

Mark Twain

HEAT CRAMPS

HEAT cramps are severe muscle cramps brought on by heat conditions and are possibly an early sign of dehydration. They can affect a person's ability to perform physical activities, like the safe operation of a motorcycle.

SIGNS and symptoms:
- o Painful involuntary muscle spasms or cramps
- o Arms, legs (especially calves), abdomen, and back muscles most effected
- o More prolonged and painful than nighttime leg cramps

DO:
- o Cool down
- o Rest
- o Drink water or sports drinks
- o Gentle stretching, gentle massage, firm pressure on cramping muscles

DON'T:
- o **Return to any strenuous use of mus: les for a few hours**
- o **Drink : arbonated, : affeinated, sweetened, or al: oholi: drinks**
- o **Ignore – : ould be a sign of impending dehydration or heat exhaustion**
- o **Take salt tablets**

SUNBURN

SUNBURN can range from a mild irritant to a serious condition. Aside from the pain and inconvenience it causes, sunburn can contribute to more serious conditions by interfering with the body's ability to effectively regulate heat.

SIGNS and symptoms:
- o Redness
- o Swelling
- o Blistering
- o Headache
- o Fever
- o Fatigue

DO:
- o Cool off in a bath or shower or by sponging off with a cool wet towel, sponge, etc.
- o Apply aloe vera lotion if available
- o Take over-the-counter pain reliever
- o Use sunblock to prevent further burning
- o Apply antibacterial ointment to blisters if they open , then cover loosely with sterile bandage
- o See your doctor if any itching or fever occur

DON'T:
- o Open blisters – leave them inta:t
- o Expose to further sun
- o Ignore – :an :ontribute to more serious :onditions

He who would travel happily must travel light.

Antoine de Saint-Exupery

DEHYDRATION

DEHYDRATION is when body fluid is lost from sweating, vomiting, or diarrhea and fluid replacement is inadequate. Dehydration can be a precursor to more serious conditions and should not be ignored.

SIGNS and symptoms:
- o Thirst – if you're thirsty you're already dehydrated
- o Dizziness, lightheadedness, or fainting
- o Weak, lethargic, or irritable
- o Difficulty thinking clearly
- o Dry or sticky mouth
- o Nausea
- o Profuse sweating
- o Dark, concentrated urine

DO:
- o Drink plenty of water before any symptoms appear
- o Drink sports drinks containing electrolytes
- o Drink small amounts frequently
- o Cool off out of the sun in shade or cool area
- o Lie down if feeling dizzy or fainting

DON'T:
- o Drink : offee or : affeinated drinks
- o Drink : arbonated drinks, or drinks with sugar or salt
- o Drink i: ed drinks – only : ool drinks
- o Drink al:ohol
- o Take salt tablets
- o Ignore symptoms, : an lead to more serious : onditions

Travel is fatal to prejudice, bigotry, and narrow mindedness, and many of our people need it sorely on these accounts. Broad, wholesome, charitable views of men and things cannot be acquired by vegetating in one little corner of the earth all one's lifetime.

Mark Twain

HEAT EXHAUSTION

HEAT exhaustion is a serious condition that can result in circulatory collapse and unconsciousness. It usually happens after repeated periods of heat exposure and fluid loss over a period of days with inadequate fluid replacement. If not treated quickly, it can develop into a life threatening situation. Proper hydration is the key to avoiding heat exhaustion.

SIGNS and symptoms:
- o Feeling faint or dizzy
- o Weakness, exhaustion, or fatigue
- o Agitated or disoriented
- o Nausea, vomiting
- o Headache
- o Pale, ashen, or gray appearance
- o Rapid heartbeat
- o Cool, moist skin or profuse sweating
- o Dilated (big) pupils
- o Thirsty
- o Slightly below normal to slightly above normal body temperature

DO:
- o Get out of the sun into shady or air conditioned area
- o Lie down, elevate feet slightly, treat for shock
- o Loosen clothing, remove whatever clothing you can

o Drink cool, not iced, water or non-sweetened sports drinks
o Spray with cool, not cold, water or sponge off with cool water, especially the head
o If high fever (especially 104 or higher), fainting, or seizures develop – call for emergency medical assistance immediately

DON'T:
o **Drink i: ed, : arbonated, : affeinated, sweetened, or al: oholi: drinks**
o **Use rubbing al: ohol to : ool**
o **Ignore it – : an be: ome life-threatening**

Thanks to the Interstate Highway System, it is now possible to travel from coast to coast without seeing anything.

Charles Kurault

HEAT STROKE

HEAT stroke, also called sunstroke, is a life threatening emergency and requires immediate emergency medical attention. Rapid treatment is critical. Heat stroke occurs when the body's heat-regulating mechanisms fail and the body generates more heat than it can dissipate. This can raise the core temperature to a life-threatening level.

SIGNS and symptoms:
- o Extremely high body temperature – 104 or higher
- o Severe changes in mental status, including irritability, confusion, disorientation, argumentativeness, or combativeness
- o Can be unconscious or in a coma-like state
- o Skin is <u>hot, red, and dry</u>
- o Absence of sweating
- o Rapid but weak pulse, can be above 160
- o Severe headache
- o Dizziness or fainting

DO:
- o Get immediate emergency medical attention – this is a life-threatening condition
- o Move into shade or air conditioning
- o Cool by sponging or spraying cool water and fanning, placing in cool bath, etc.
- o Lie down, elevate feet, treat for shock

o Apply cold packs to neck, armpits, and groin areas

DON'T:
- o **Give <u>any</u> fluids – <u>espe: ially</u> alcohol, iced drinks, or caffeinated drinks**
- o **Apply rubbing alcohol**
- o **Give salt tablets**
- o **Forget to summon emergency medical attention immediately**

You're the guy that'll be sneaking out of your bedroom at three o'clock in the morning to look at your bike.

Paul Teutul Sr.

PART 4

TRAUMA

THE most obvious cause of trauma for motorcyclists is, of course, collision with another vehicle or stationary object. It is of little consequence to the injured victim if the collision was caused by that idiot in the car turning left in front of them or because they were just going too fast around that corner or didn't notice that puddle of diesel fuel. Even when we have done everything possible to prevent situations that can lead to accidents and the resulting trauma, sometimes things happen that are out of our control. Thankfully, the results of the majority of these incidents will be minor, and can be handled effectively with first aid. Knowing what to do, being able to do it quickly, and having the right tools to do it can many times make the difference between being able to successfully and safely complete the ride or not, and may have a profound effect on the victim's recovery and rehabilitation from the injury.

ONE of the most important things to remember at any motorcycle accident is that many times the injured victim will ignore or minimize their injuries. This can result in much more serious consequences than had the injury been appropriately attended to from the beginning. With all of the adrenalin and confusion at any accident scene it is critical that someone calmly and accurately assess everyone involved in the accident. Head, neck, spinal, and internal injuries can be less than obvious and should be suspected in every motorcycle accident. If there is any question or doubt at all about the presence of or the severity of any injury, emergency medical services should be called immediately. It is always better to be safe than sorry.

Patience is something you admire in the driver behind you and scorn in the one ahead.

Mac McCleary

SHOCK

SHOCK is a very serious medical condition that can affect anyone at an accident. Everyone at an accident scene should be evaluated for possible shock. Shock may be the result of trauma, loss of blood or internal bleeding, heatstroke, allergic reaction, or other conditions like infection or poisoning. A person in shock may not appear to have any injuries and may deny having the symptoms of shock.

SIGNS and symptoms of shock:
- o Cool, clammy skin may appear gray or pale
- o Pulse is rapid but weak
- o Breathing may be rapid or slow and shallow
- o Pupils may be dilated
- o Person may feel weak
- o May appear confused, overly exited, anxious, or have a 'spacey' or vacant look

DO:
- o Lie down flat with feet slightly elevated
- o Keep calm and still
- o Keep warm (not hot), cover with a blanket, jacket, or whatever is available
- o Turn them on their side if vomiting or bleeding from the mouth

DON'T:

o   **Give anything to eat or drink, even water**

I believe many Harley guys spend more time revving their engines than actually driving anywhere; I sometimes wonder why they bother to have wheels on their motorcycles.

Dave Barry

BLEEDING

UNCONTOLLED excessive bleeding can very quickly become a life-threatening situation, so it is extremely important to recognize and effectively attend to this condition immediately.

SIGNS and symptoms:
- o A large amount of blood spurting or flowing from a wound, or a smaller amount that does not stop

DO:
- o Lie the person down with their head slightly lower than their body or elevate their legs to increase the blood flow to the brain
- o Elevate the area of bleeding if possible
- o Remove any obvious easily-removable debris from the bleeding site
- o Apply direct pressure to the bleeding site with bandage, cloth, piece of clothing, or your hand if nothing else is available. Ideally, use a sterile non stick bandage if available
- o Maintain pressure until bleeding completely stops, at least 20 – 30 minutes
- o When the bleeding stops, bind the wound firmly but not over-tightly with a bandage, cloth, or clothing and adhesive tape or elastic bandage

- o If bleeding doesn't slow with pressure, squeeze or apply pressure to the main artery feeding blood to that area –
- o Arm – inside of the arm just above   the elbow or just below the arm pit
- o Leg – behind the knee or in the groin
- o Continue applying direct pressure to the wound while applying pressure to the pressure point
- o Seek immediate emergency medical attention if you suspect internal bleeding, any bleeding from body cavities (ears, nose, rectum, etc), vomiting or coughing up blood, any immediate bruising on neck, chest or abdomen, any wounds that have penetrated the head, chest, or abdomen, and for any suspicions of fractures and shock

DON'T:
- o **Remove large or deeply imbedded obje: ts**
- o **Probe the wound**
- o **Attempt to : lean the wound or remove the bandage before the bleeding is stopped - add more absorbent material on top of it if needed**

MINOR CUTS & SCRAPES

SIMPLE wounds, small cuts, and scrapes usually don't require emergency medical care but should be treated properly to avoid infection or other serious complications.

SIGNS and symptoms:
- o   Small open wound
- o   Little to moderate bleeding

DO:
- o   Stop the bleeding by applying direct pressure to the wound with a clean cloth or sterile bandage
- o   Clean the wound by rinsing with clean or sterile water
- o   Use sterilized tweezers to remove dirt/debris after rinsing
- o   Apply antibiotic cream after the bleeding has stopped
- o   Cover the wound lightly with a non-stick bandage
- o   For deeper cuts use butterfly bandages to hold the cut closed
- o   Seek immediate medical attention if the blood spurts or does not stop flowing after 20 – 30 minutes of direct pressure
- o   See your doctor if there is any redness, drainage, swelling, or warmth
- o   See your doctor ASAP about a tetanus shot

DON'T:
- o Keep : he: king to see if the bleeding has stopped – : he: k after 20 – 30 minutes of dire:t pr essure
- o Use soap dire: tly on the wound – only around it
- o Apply hydrogen peroxide or iodine dire: tly to wound
- o Apply pressure with gauze – it will sti: k to the wound
- o Tou: h the wound with your hand

Unusual travel suggestions are dancing lessons from God.

Kurt Vonnegut

FINGERTIP AVULSION

STICKING your fingers into running machinery may not sound like a smart thing to do, but is a frequent occurrence for motorcyclists trying to diagnose or fix an errant motorcycle. Also, sliding along asphalt can grind away unprotected body parts, like the tips of your fingers.

SIGNS and symptoms:
- o   The tip of the finger cut or pinched off or ground down
- o   Pain, bleeding, or other unpleasantness

DO:
- o   Apply antibiotic cream to wound
- o   Apply non-stick dressing   with gentle compression and
- o   Use a small gauze pad on the end of the finger and
- o   Cover with fingertip bandage or
- o   Cut out L-shaped gauze (see illustration), place short leg of gauze over fingertip and wrap the longer leg around the finger then secure with tape
- o   Seek medical attention ASAP

DON'T:
- o   **Wrap gauze or tape too tightly around finger, it may a:t as a tourniquet and restri:t blood flow to the finger**

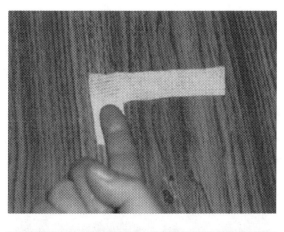

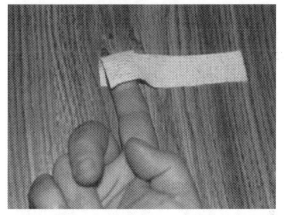

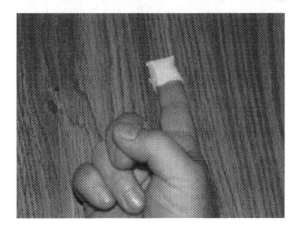

AVULSED FINGER/TOENAIL

STICKING fingers into running machinery can sometimes be explained, but getting a toenail ripped off will probably happen in an off-bike moment, assuming the motorcyclist wears shoes while riding. Stranger things have happened.

SIGNS and symptoms:
- o A toe or finger nail that is completely torn off or may be partially attached
- o A nail completely torn off with an exposed nail bed may appear as if the nail is still in place
- o Pain, tenderness, possibly bleeding

DO:
- o Cleanse thoroughly with room temperature saline or sterile water
- o Apply antibiotic cream
- o Leave the nail in place if possible
- o Apply non-stick dressing

DON'T:
- o **Apply ordinary gauze dressing – will adhere and : ause pain when removed**
- o **Try to rip off a dangling nail – try to se: ure it in pla: e**

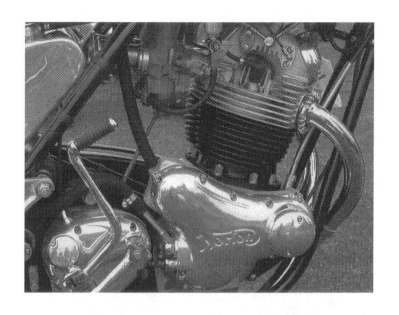

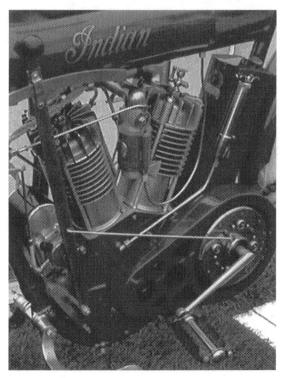

ROAD RASH

ROAD RASH, also called trauma tattoo, is all too often the result of a motorcyclist's intimate encounter with their immediate environment, particularly the road   they ride on. The better the riding gear you use, the less road rash you will have to deal with if you have one of those intimate encounters with the road.

SIGNS and symptoms: The severity of road rash can be graded similar to that of burns:
- o First degree – only the skin surface is reddened
- o Second degree – the surface layer is broken or abraded but the deeper layer is intact
- o Third degree – the skin is entirely abraded through to the underlying layer of fat, tissue, etc.
- o Road debris is usually imbedded in the abrasion
- o Some skin fragments may be hanging loose

DO: The goal is to keep the road rash clean, infection-free, and moist to prevent scab formation allowing it to heal from the bottom up and the edges in
- o Clean the wound thoroughly by flushing with saline solution or clean, clear skin temperature water

- o Applying Bacitracin or other antibiotic ointment prior to cleaning may help loosen tar, grease, or other debris from the wound
- o Use a new or sterilized toothbrush to **very gently** scrub away dirt and debris while flooding with saline solution or water– you must be very careful not to further damage the area by scrubbing too vigorously
- o Larger pieces of debris can be removed with sterilized tweezers
- o Small pieces of skin hanging from the edges can be cut with sterilized scissors, but not large chunks of skin
- o When the rash has been thoroughly cleaned, apply an antibiotic ointment and cover with one of the following:
  - o Vaseline gauze
  - o Hydrocolloidal dressing such as Duoderm to absorb exudate
  - o Semi–occlusive dressing such as Bioclusive or Tegaderm to evaporate exudate

DON'T:
- o **Cleanse with antisepti: s like al: ohol, povidone-iodine, or hydrogen peroxide whi: h : an : ause further tissue damage and slow the healing pro: ess**
- o **Flush with water that is hotter or : older than body temperature whi: h : an be painful to the sensitive abrasion**
- o **Cover with a dressing that will sti: k**
- o **Expose to sun or allow to sunburn**

PUNCTURE WOUNDS

A PUNCTURE wound is whenever something pierces the skin rather than cuts it, causing a smaller, deeper wound. Falling down on a motorcycle or running into something frequently results in something unwanted puncturing our body. If the object causing the puncture remains imbedded, it is an impalement rather than a simple puncture.

SIGNS and symptoms:
- o Doesn't usually cause excessive bleeding
- o The wound may seem to close immediately on its own
- o If the object causing the puncture remains in the skin, see the section on "Foreign Object In The Skin"
- o Infection and tetanus are two major concerns for this injury
- o If there is excessive bleeding, see the section on "Bleeding"

DO:
- o If there is minor bleeding, let it bleed a while to help clean itself out
- o If minor bleeding doesn't stop on its own, apply gentle, direct pressure with a clean bandage or cloth
- o Remove only small loose debris
- o Apply antibiotic cream

o Cover the wound with a loose non-stick bandage
o See your doctor immediately about a tetanus shot, if there is persistent or excessive bleeding, if there is an object imbedded in the wound, or if you see any signs of infection

DON'T:
o **Remove any large imbedded obje:ts or any obje:ts if there is ex:essive bleeding or gushing blood**

I'd rather be riding my motorcycle and thinking about God than sitting in church and thinking about riding my motorcycle.

Anonymous

BLUNT SCROTAL TRAUMA

BLUNT scrotal trauma obviously can only affect the male portion of the motorcycling population, but those affected will certainly know it. Gas tanks and other hard parts can be a source of great pain when our machines come to a stop quicker than our bodies do.

SIGNS and symptoms:
- o Intense pain
- o Bruising
- o Swelling
- o Scrotum may appear empty if there is testicular dislocation (testis may be inside the abdominal wall)
- o Testes may appear 'deformed' or of abnormal shape if ruptured

DO:
- o Apply cold pack or ice pack
- o Take aspirin or other pain reliever
- o Seek immediate emergency medical attention if unable to urinate, any bloody discharge or bloody urine, or any dislocation or rupture of testes
- o If you are going to be waiting awhile before continuing your ride (a good idea) or once you get home, apply a scrotal support (see illustration)

DON'T:

- o Leave the i:e pa:k or :old pa:k on too long or apply i:e dire:tly to the skin, :an :ause ti ssue damage
- o Pi:k this time to get amorous

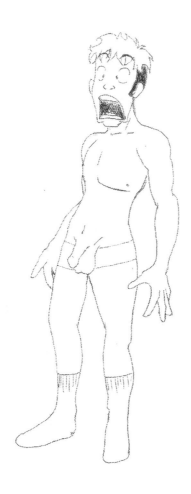

BRUISES

BRUISES form when small blood vessels near the surface of the skin rupture releasing blood out underneath the skin usually from a blow or bump.

SIGNS and symptoms:
- o Black and blue marks
- o Tiny red dots or red splotches
- o Pain or tenderness

DO:
- o Elevate the area if possible
- o Apply ice or cold pack
- o Take over the counter pain relievers
- o See your Doctor if accompanied by excessive persistent pain or headache, or abnormal or excessive bleeding elsewhere

DON'T:
- o **Apply a bandage if the skin is not broken**
- o **Leave i: e or : old pa: k on long enough to :ause ti ssue damage**

DENTAL FRACTURE

RATHER than a tooth that's been knocked out, this is when a tooth has been broken off, or when there has been a simple fracture of the tooth exposing dentin without breaking off any of the tooth.

SIGNS and symptoms:
- o Exposed dentin (yellow pulpy stuff)
- o Possible bleeding
- o Pain
- o Could indicate a fractured jaw if several teeth feel loose and move together

DO:
- o Avoid hot or cold food or drinks
- o If fractured but not broken off, the exposed fracture on the tooth can be covered with nail polish to temporarily protect it
- o Exposed pulp can be covered with moist cotton
- o Give aspirin, Tylenol, or Motrin for pain
- o Seek professional dental care ASAP

DON'T:
- o **Overlook the possibility of a jaw or fa: ial fra: ture**
- o **Overlook the possibility of a ne: k injury**

AVULSED TOOTH

RUNNING into stationary objects with your face can have some unwanted and painful results. Sometimes running one's mouth off and getting punched in the mouth can have the same results – teeth that used to be in your mouth but aren't there anymore.

SIGNS and symptoms:
- o Whole teeth that are knocked out, not broken off
- o Pain
- o Possible bleeding

DO:
- o Use a tooth storage device (such as 'Save A Tooth') available from a dentist, pharmacy, or medical supply store, if you have one in your first aid kit
- o Handle the tooth only by the top, not the root
- o Rinse the tooth with clean, clear or sterile warm water
- o Try to replace it in the socket right away, then bite down on a gauze roll or cloth to help keep it in place and possibly re-seat it
- o If you can't replace it in the socket, store it in warm salt water, warm milk, or your own saliva
- o Get medical or dental attention ASAP

DON'T:

- o **Rub or s: rape the tooth to remove dirt or debris from it**
- o **Hold the tooth under running water, put it in a :u p or bowl instead**

Your road is everything that a road ought to be... and yet you will not stay on it half a mile, for the reason that little, seductive, mysterious roads are always branching out from it on either hand, and as these curve sharply also and hide what is beyond, you cannot resist the temptation to desert your own chosen road and explore them.

Mark Twain

SPRAINS

A SPRAIN is an injury to a ligament, which is the tough elastic tissue attached to a person's bones holding their joints in place.   The ligament can be over-stretched, torn, or completely detached.

SIGNS and symptoms:
- o   Rapid swelling and pain
- o   Usually in the ankles, knees, elbows, wrists, or arches of the feet
- o   The greater the pain the more severe the injury

DO:
- o   Apply ice to the area to reduce swelling and pain
- o   If ice is not available, use cold water
- o   Compress the area with an elastic wrap or bandage
- o   Rest the injured limb and protect with a splint if possible
- o   Elevate the injured limb if possible
- o   Summon emergency medical assistance if there was a 'popping' sound or if there is extreme pain

DON'T:
- o   **Apply i: e dire: tly to skin or leave i: e on too long, : an : ause tissue damage**

DISLOCATIONS

DISLOCATIONS are when the bones are forced from their natural position in the joints; usually in the fingers, elbows, shoulders, knees, kneecaps, toes, and sometimes in the jaw, hip or ankle.

SIGNS and symptoms:
- o Usually a very obvious deformity of the joint
- o Sudden intense sharp pain
- o Immobilization of the joint

DO:
- o Splint the affected joint in the position it is in to prevent any movement of the joint
- o Apply ice or cold pack to reduce swelling and control internal bleeding
- o Use a sling for arms
- o Tape fingers or toes together to stabilize if possible
- o Get immediate medical attention
- o Give pain medication

DON'T:
- o **Move the joint or attempt to put it ba: k in pla: e**

FRACTURES

FRACTURES are broken bones. The break can range from a simple crack in the bone to a complete break. The worst fracture is a complete break and dislocation of the broken bones that pierces the skin (compound fracture). In this case, one of the major concerns is the broken bones severing blood vessels, causing serious internal or external bleeding.

SIGNS and symptoms:
- o The limb appears deformed or at an unnatural angle
- o Possible bleeding
- o Bone may have pierced the skin
- o Gentle pressure or any movement causes intense pain

DO:
- o Stop any excessive bleeding by applying direct pressure on the wound site with a gauze pad, cloth, etc until the bleeding stops
- o Immobilize the area by splinting (see below) to prevent any movement
- o Treat for shock if the person is faint or if there is any difficulty breathing
- o Seek immediate medical attention

DON'T:

> o **Try to re-align the bones ba:k into their proper position**

PROPER SPLINTING:

Moldable soft metal splinting devices, like a Sam Splint or an aluminum wire splint, are very effective and can be rolled up small enough to be carried in a kit. If you do not have one of these, use something rigid, preferably metal, wood, or hard plastic, that is longer than the bone being immobilized so that it extends above and below the break to immobilize and prevent any movement of the break. Pad the splint with gauze, cloth, etc. Attach the splint to the broken limb with gauze, cloth, an Ace wrap, or even a belt, tight enough to prevent movement but not tight enough to restrict blood flow. Even a magazine rolled around an arm or   leg   and secured with a belt or ace wrap can be an effective splint. Legs, fingers, or toes may sometimes be splinted together to prevent movement. The whole idea is that the less movement of the break, the better.

NOSE FRACTURE

FRACTURED noses are usually the result of running nose-first into some immoveable object or, sometimes, from sticking that nose where it doesn't belong. Either way, it hurts.

SIGNS and symptoms:
- o Swelling and tenderness of the nose
- o Usually has minimal bleeding
- o Possible deformation of the nose
- o Possible difficulty breathing through the nose

DO:
- o Apply ice or cold packs
- o Pack the nose with gauze if there is any bleeding that doesn't stop
- o Seek medical attention ASAP

DON'T:
- o **Attempt to 'reposition' a displa: ed nose**
- o **Pa: k the nose with gauze if the bleeding stops or is minor**

Safety doesn't happen by accident.

Anonymous

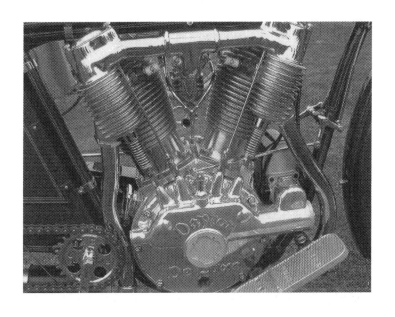

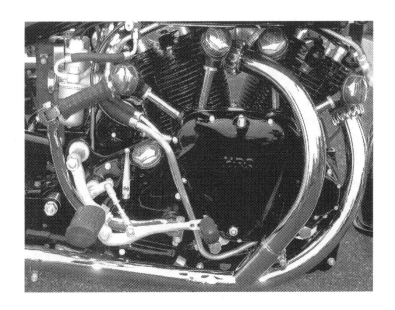

HEAD INJURY

HEAD INJURY is a major concern for motorcyclists. Motor vehicle accidents, including motorcycles, are the leading cause of head injuries in general and fatal head injuries in particular. The quicker a head injury is identified and interventions started, the better the chance for survival and minimal disability. Remember that symptoms from a head injury causing bleeding in the brain can be delayed 24 hours or more.

SIGNS and symptoms:
- o Loss of consciousness or change in level of consciousness
- o Convulsions
- o Confusion, loss of balance, slurred speech
- o Drowsiness or lethargy
- o Weakness in or inability to use arms or legs
- o Unequal pupil size
- o Vomiting
- o Bleeding from the head or facial area, especially the mouth, nose, or ears
- o Bruising behind the ears or under the eyes
- o Headache
- o Lack of vital signs (breathing and heartbeat)

DO:
- o Summon emergency medical services immediately

o   Have the person lie down and remain still until help arrives – sometimes people with head injuries don't realize they are seriously injured
o   If there is any excessive bleeding, apply direct pressure with gauze pad, cloth, etc
o   If there is a suspicion of a neck injury, stabilize the neck, head, and shoulders
o   Check for breathing and pulse – start CPR if needed

DON'T:
o   **Give the person anything to eat or drink**
o   **Elevate the feet**
o   **Give any pain medi: ation**
o   **Remove their helmet unless there is bleeding from the head or CPR is needed (see se: tion on "A: : ident S: ene Management" for information on removing a helmet when ne: essary)**

Get a 'cycle.   You won't regret it.   If you live.

Mark Twain

CERVICAL / SPINAL INJURIES

NECK AND BACK injuries can end a riding career (or a life) in the blink of an eye. Good riding gear with back armor can make a critical difference in many motorcycling accidents, and every motorcyclist should seriously consider the level of risk versus the cost/comfort/fashion considerations when deciding what gear they will use.

SIGNS and symptoms:
- o Severe pain in neck or back
- o Unable to move neck, arms, or legs
- o Neck or back is twisted or at an odd angle
- o Weakness, numbness, or paralysis
- o Loss of bladder or bowel control

DO:
- o Summon EMS immediately
- o Have the person lie still and keep movement to a minimum
- o Use rolled up jackets or clothing to hold the head/neck/back in position
- o Check for vital signs (breathing and pulse)

DON'T:
- o Remove their helmet unless ne: essary for CPR or to stop bleeding (see se: tion on A:: ident S: ene Management for instru: tions on removing helmet)
- o Move the person unless ne: essary

Well trained reflexes are quicker than luck.

Anonymous

Appendix

SKILLS IMPROVEMENT

It is known that the vast majority of single vehicle motorcycle accidents happen on curves. Whether it is because of hazards in the roadway (sand, water, oil, diesel fuel, etc.) or simply because the rider was going faster than his skill would allow is not known. Personal experience and talking with many motorcycle riders would indicate that many times a rider loses it in the middle of a turn by not knowing or executing good cornering skills, or simply by freaking out and doing the wrong thing. This is something that can be greatly improved by education and practice. Below is a list of street-oriented riding classes that any rider can benefit from.

> Motorcycle Safety Foundation
> Beginner and Experienced Rider courses
> www.msf-usa.org
> Phone #   800-446-9227
>
> StreetMasters Cornering Workshops
> Advanced cornering skills for the street done on the safety of a track
> www.streetmasters.info
> Phone#   805-464-0544

Lee Parks Advanced Riding Clinic
Excellant advanced skills class
www.totalcontroltraining.net
Phone #   800-943-5638

FIRST AID KITS

THE first rule of First Aid Kits is "Let the Context Dictate the Contents." In other words, what you need is determined by what you are going to do with it. There are many excellent First Aid Kits on the market today. Although there are many choices in style and content, the needs of motorcyclists are specific enough to require a kit purposefully designed for motorcyclists, so you will probably need to 'customize' a manufactured kit or build your own. The usefulness of any toolkit depends on having the tools you need without carrying a lot of stuff you probably won't use.

WITH this in mind, we need to assemble our first aid kit with the tools needed to address the most common environmental and trauma injuries motorcyclists are subject to. The following is a list of suggested equipment, hardware, and supplies derived from the injuries addressed in this manual and can be used to assemble anything from a small basic kit to a complete kit able to address any emergency.

CARRYING DEVICE: a hard weather-proof case or soft-case with supplies in zip-lock bags to protect contents from exposure to rain, etc.

WOUND CARE: one of the most-used parts of the kit
- o 4x4 or 3x3 gauze pads
- o non-stick dressings/Telfa pads
- o 8x7 combine dressing
- o 3″ or 4″ occlusive dressing (Tegaderm, Biocclusive)
- o hydrocolloidal dressing (Duoderm)
- o band-aids (small, large, fingertip, knuckle, butterfly)
- o cloth tape
- o duct tape
- o roller gauze
- o sterile eye pad
- o medical scrub/cleansing soap

MEDICATIONS: over-the-counter meds & any personal prescription meds
- o antibiotic-cream/Neosporin/triple antibiotic cream
- o Tylenol/Motrin/aspirin
- o Benadryl/Sudafed/antihistimine
- o Ora-gel/Orabase
- o Tinactin/Mycostatin/anti-fungal cream
- o Hydrocortisone cream

HARDWARE:
- o tweezers
- o safety pins
- o plastic bags
- o thermometer/Tempa-dots
- o scissors
- o 60cc irrigation syringe / squirtable bottle

o Sam splint/aluminum wire splint
o New toothbrush (in factory-sealed container)

MISCELLANEOUS:
o latex/plastic exam gloves
o CPR pocket mask
o red plastic bags
o hot/cold packs
o space blanket/survival blanket
o mineral oil
o antiseptic/alcohol towelettes
o Q-tips
o Save-a-Tooth container
o Hand sanitizer/Purell
o sterile saline
o Ace wrap/Coban/Kling
o Triangle bandage/sling
o moleskin/molefoam
o eyewash kit

REFERENCES

The following are good research references to read for anyone wanting to get real information on any of these subjects or who wants to be able to speak knowledgably about any of this:

o Bigelow, 9 . (2001). *Traumatic Brain Injury Associated with Motorcycle Crashes in Wisconsin, 1991-1997.* Paper Presented at the International Motorcycle Safety Conference, Orlando, Florida.

o Center for Urban Transportation Research (1998). 1998 Florida Observational Motorcycle Helmet Use Study. Tampa: University of South Florida.

o Finison, K.S. (2001). Using CODES Linked Data to Evaluate Motorcycle Crashes in Maine. Paper Presented at the International Motorcycle Safety Conference, Orlando, Florida.

o Fleming, H.S. and Becker, E.R. (1992). The impact of the Texas 1989 motorcycle helmet law on total and head-related fatalities, severe injuries, and overall injuries. Medical Care, 30, 832-845.

o Gabella, B., Reiner, K.L., Hoffman, R.E., Cook, M. and Stallones, L. (1995).

Relationship of helmet use and head injuries among motorcycle crash victims in El Paso County, Colorado, 1989-1990. Accident Analysis and Prevention, 27, 363-369

o Hotz, G.A., Cohn, S.M., Popkin, B.A., Ekeh, P., Duncan, R., Johnson, E.W., Pernas, F. and Selem, J. (2002). The impact of a repealed motorcycle helmet law in Miami-Dade County. The Journal of Trauma, Injury, Infection, and Critical Care, 52, 469-474.

o Kelley, P., Sanson, T., Strange, G. and Orsay, E. (1991). A prospective study of the impact of helmet usage on motorcycle trauma. Annals of Emergency Medicine, 20, 852-856.

o Kraus, J.F. and Peek, C. (1995). The impact of two related prevention strategies on head injury reduction among non-fatally injured motorcycle riders, California, 1991-1993. Journal of Neurotrauma, 12, 873-881.

o Kraus, J.F., Peek, C., McArthur, D.L., and Williams, A. (1994). The effect of the 1992 California motorcycle helmet usage law on motorcycle crash fatalities and injuries. JAMA, 272, 1506-1511.

o Kraus, J.F., Peek, C., Shen, H. and 9 illiams, A. (1995). Motorcycle crashes: injuries, rider, crash and vehicle characteristics associated with helmet use. Journal of Traffic Medicine, 23, 29-35.

o Max, 9 ., Stark B., and Root, S. (1998). Putting a lid on injury costs: The economic impact of the California Motorcycle Helmet Law. Journal of Trauma, Injury, Infection and Critical Care, 45, 550-556.

o Mitchell, K.A., Kufera, J.A., Ballesteros, M.F., Smialek, J.E., and Dischinger, P.C. (2001). Autopsy Study of Motorcyclist Fatalities: The Effect of the 1992 Maryland Helmet Use Law. Paper Presented at the International Motorcycle Safety Conference, Orlando, Florida.

o Mock, C.N., Maier, R.V., Boyle, E., Pilcher, S. and Rivara, F.P. (1995). Injury prevention strategies to promote helmet use decrease severe head injuries at a Level 1 trauma center. Journal of Trauma, 39, 29-35.

o Muller, A. (2004). Florida's motorcycle helmet law repeal and fatality rates. American Journal of Public Health, 94, 556-558.

o   Preusser, F.F., Hedlund, J.H. and Ulmer, R.G. (2000). Evaluation of Motorcycle Helmet Law Repeal in Arkansas and Texas. DOT HS 80W131. Washington DC: U.S. Department of Transportation.

o   Rowland, J., Rivara, F.P., Salzberg, P., Soderberg, R., Maier, R.V. and Koepsell, T. (1W6). Motorcycle helmet use and injury outcome and hospitalization costs from crashes in Washington state. American Journal of Public Health, 86, 41-45.

o   Rutledge, R. and Stutts, J. (1W3). The association of helmet use with the outcome of motorcycle crash injury when controlling for crash/injury severity. Accident Analysis and Prevention, 25, 347-353.

o   Sarkar, S., Peek, C. and Kraus, J.F. (1W5). Fatal injuries in motorcycle riders according to helmet use. Journal of Trauma, 38, 242-245.

o   Shankar, B.S., Ramzy, A.I., Soderstrom, C.A., Dischinger, P.C. and Clark, C.C. (1W2). Helmet use, patterns of injury, medial outcome, and costs among motorcycle drivers in Maryland. Accident Analysis and Prevention, 24, 385-3W6.

o Shankar, U. (2001). Fatal Single Vehicle Motorcycle Crashes DOT HS 80W360. Washington DC: U.S. Department of Transportation.

o Shankar, U. (2001). Motorcyclist Fatalities in 2000. DOT HS 80W387. Washington DC: U.S. Department of Transportation.

o Shankar, U. (2001). Recent Trends in Fatal Motorcycle Crashes. DOT HS 80W271. Washington DC: U.S. Department of Transportation

o Stolzenberg, L. and D'Alessio, S.J. (2003). "Born to be wild" The effect of the repeal of Florida's mandatory motorcycle helmet-use law on serious injury and fatality rates. Evaluation Review, 27, 131-150.

o Traffic Tech Technology Transfer Series, Number 127, June 1WW. National Public Services Research Institute "Do Motorcycle Helmets Interfere with the Vision and Hearing of Riders?"

o Ulmer, R., and Northrup, V.S. (2005). Evaluation of the Repeal of the All-Rider Motorcycle Helmet Law in Florida. Washington DC: U.S. Department of Transportation.

o Ulmer, R.G. and Preusser, D.F. (2003). Evaluation of the Repeal of Motorcycle Helmet Laws in Kentucky and Louisiana. DOT HS 80W 530. Washington DC: National Highway Traffic Safety Administration.